8·7·78

MULTIPLE SCLEROSIS
SCARS OF CHILDHOOD
New Horizons and Hope

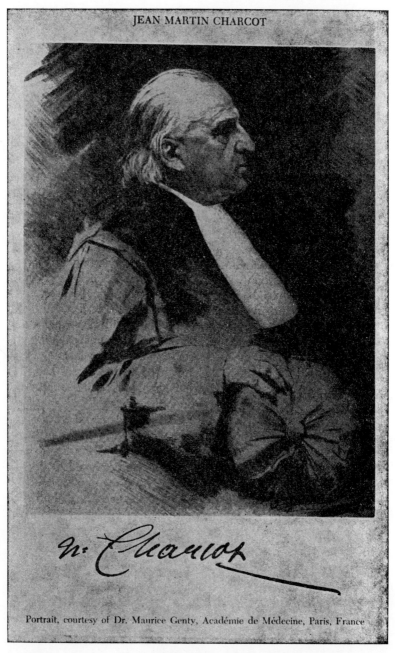

Portrait, courtesy of Dr. Maurice Genty, Académie de Médecine, Paris, France

Jean Martin Charcot

Jean Martin Charcot (1825-1893) was born in Paris, the son of a carriage builder. Charcot had both industry and curiosity. He became a great neuropathologist; as a clinician he was even greater. His description of disseminated (multiple) sclerosis embodied the three classic signs and symptoms, tremor, nystagmus and scanning speech. He was the most colorful teacher of medicine of his day.

MULTIPLE SCLEROSIS

SCARS OF CHILDHOOD

New Horizons and Hope

By

John M. Adams, M.D., Ph.D.

Professor of Pediatrics, Emeritus
School of Medicine
University of California
Los Angeles

With a Foreword by

ROBERT A. GOOD, Ph.D., M.D.
President and Director
Sloan-Kettering Institute for Cancer Research
New York

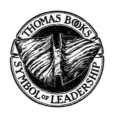

CHARLES C THOMAS · PUBLISHER
Springfield · Illinois · U.S.A.

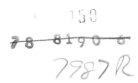

Published and Distributed Throughout the World by
CHARLES C THOMAS • PUBLISHER
Bannerstone House
301-327 East Lawrence Avenue, Springfield, Illinois, U.S.A.

© 1977, by CHARLES C THOMAS • PUBLISHER
ISBN 0-398-03595-4
Library of Congress Catalog Card Number: 76-21625

Printed in the United States of America
W-2

Library of Congress Cataloging in Publication Data

Adams, John Milton, 1905-
    MS, scars of childhood.
    Multiple Sclerosis, scars of childhood.

    Includes index.
    1. Multiple sclerosis.   I.   Title.
RC377.A33   616.8'34   76-21625
ISBN 0-398-03595-4

PREFACE

Doctor Adams, does anyone know what causes MS? Why did I get MS while none of my family or friends got it? Is there a drug to stabilize MS? Can MS be prevented? I hear on television and radio and read in magazines about 'viruses,' 'immunity,' 'interferon' and more recently, about 'transfer factor.' What do these words mean and what do they have to do with MS?"

These are some of the questions MS patients and their families have asked me over the several years I have been attending MS clinics. In answering their questions I have come to realize that there must be many other MS patients and members of their families who have a keen interest in MS and especially how it affects them.

I have written this small book to tell the story of MS as I tell it to my patients—as clearly and concisely as I can. Some rather complex subjects cannot be covered simply. A glossary with definitions of the less familiar words has been included but even with the help of definitions there may be words, phrases, whole sentences and, perhaps, chapters you will not understand. These you may wish to discuss with your doctor.

Although this book was written primarily for MS patients, their families and friends, there is much in it that is new and should be of interest to nurses, occupational and physical therapists and general physicians, all of whom may be involved in the care of MS patients.

This book has been titled "Multiple Sclerosis—Scars of Childhood" because there is evidence that the disease starts years before the first symptoms appear, most likely in childhood. There also is increasing evidence that "scars" are the result of damage caused by viruses of such common contagious disease of children as measles, chicken pox or smallpox vaccination. These viruses may persist in certain cells in the body for months or years before they cause disease. Another disease that is similar to MS in the kind of scarring to the brain, called SSPE (subacute sclerosing panencephalitis) has been proved to be caused by measles virus.

This book is a compilation of chapters about subjects related in one way or another to MS. Part I is about patients. It describes the disease and explains how it causes the symptoms and signs. It discusses exacerbations, remissions and prognosis. Part II is devoted to the progress being made in research which is opening up new horizons and offering new hope to MS patients. The deep concern for further understanding of the many unsolved problems relevant to MS is emphasized by the impressive dollar amount (exceeding $21,000,000 per year) funded for research by the National Multiple Sclerosis Society, the National Institute of Neurological and Communicative Disorders and Stroke, several Foundations and private donors. Benefits to mankind must surely come from a concentration and fusion of knowledge as it accumulates in laboratories and clinics around the world. There is hope that someday MS will no longer be one of the serious illnesses of human beings. Like poliomyelitis, rabies, and smallpox, it can conceivably be eradicated from the world.

J.M.A.

FOREWORD

I REMEMBER WELL my first meeting with John Adams in in 1945 when I was a junior medical student receiving my initial orientation to Pediatrics in Irvine McQuarrie's Department at the University of Minnesota. Already at that time, John Adams was teaching—emphasizing, and I thought sometimes overemphasizing—that common infections like measles, influenza, rubella, mumps, and vaccinia virus infection, were not as bland as we thought them to be. To him, they were certainly not the simple, annoying, common, contagious infections of childhood, but were often serious diseases the consequences and sequelae of which could be fatal or produce long-lasting, sometimes devastating illness.

Already in those early days, Adams was insisting that these common diseases, in just the right circumstances, or by infecting just the right child, could produce very serious consequences. The stage of life, the particular genetic make-up, state of nutrition, and/or state of immunologic responsiveness, he insisted, could transform these common contagions or vaccinations into the most devastating diseases of man. Some of us medical students thought Adams, with his enchantment for inclusion bodies, post-mortem examinations, and lovely experimental models, was too much obsessed with the potential hazards of childhood infections. Time has proved us wrong, and him right! Increasing evidence, derived in part from a surging technology, especially in the immunologic and virologic fields, has revealed the nature and hazard of latent and continuing virus infections; thus, dologies have been confirmed when scientists developed many of Adam's interpretations drawn from simple metho-

sophisticated techniques to address the questions he put in focus.

In this volume, written for the patient with multiple sclerosis, members of his family, nurses, social workers, and general physicians on whom much of the care of multiple sclerosis patients devolves, Dr. John Adams explains with admirable clarity the modern view of the associations between multiple sclerosis and common virus infections. Without imposing unnecessary concerns with high technology, we are given a picture of multiple sclerosis which includes its discovery, definition as a disease, and clinical picture. His simple yet accurate description gives us both an authoritative and optimistic perspective. Even some of the exciting current experimental leads that are yielding trials of new forms of treatment for multiple sclerosis are cautiously described and analysed.

I agree with Dr. Adams that continued pursuit of research efforts to define the etiology of multiple sclerosis in terms of common virus infections, that in some way go wrong and are not handled properly in some of many persons infected, promises to yield improvement in early diagnosis, bringing powerful new tools of immunotherapy, antiviral therapy and immunoprophylaxis to the conquest of multiple sclerosis. These tools in turn promise to provide substantial improvement in outlook and, ultimately, I contend, the means of prevention of this dread disease. Much challenge and several discoveries and a great deal of work lie ahead before all this can be realized, but one can think about multiple sclerosis these days with guarded optimism because of the progress Adams sees in the research in this field.

This book will offer hope in concrete terms from one who knows multiple sclerosis intimately to those who must suffer the disease, or maintain, encourage and treat its victims. It has been a pleasure for me to renew contact with my teacher of yesteryear through this book. Once again, I have learned much and have been inspired by his teaching.

ROBERT A. GOOD

INTRODUCTION

IT WAS A hundred years ago that Jean Martin Charcot (1825-1893) recorded the classical signs and symptoms of multiple sclerosis which he said were *tremor* and *nystagmus,* jerky eye movements when the patient looks to one side or the other and occasionally with upward gaze. The third symptom which he elaborated was a resitant or slow jerky type of talking called *scanning speech.* Charcot was the first to describe concisely the changes in the brain as seen by the microscope after the patient has passed away. He pointed out that the coverings of the nerves were destroyed, and he called this demyelination or a lack of myelin. At the same time the nerve itself did not appear to be harmed but continued in the presence of the scarred tissue called a *plaque.* The process of destruction affects the coverings of the nerves (myelin) first, but it also occurs in little islands or discrete areas about the veins in the brain and spinal cord. The exact mechanism by which this occurs was unknown to Charcot.

Viruses which cause common illnesses in childhood after a rather long period of silence may become active and account for higher levels of antibodies, protein substances in blood serum which interfere with the action of the viruses. The author and D. T. Imagawa (1962) found that patients with MS had high levels of *measles* antibodies in their blood serum and spinal fluid. This interference effect might explain why many patients with MS have periods when they are much better. As the interfering process wears out, recurrence of symptoms such as a decrease in vision or hearing is likely.

Dr. J. H. D. Millar (1971), a distinguished neurologist at Queens University in Belfast, Ireland, points out in his book that multiple sclerosis is a disease which often may be traced from early childhood. The symptoms may be very mild with recovery apparently taking place, or attacks become more severe and the patient develops a serious disability.

While MS may develop in childhood, it is relatively uncommon and most signs and symptoms begin between the ages of twenty and forty years. Millar also emphasized the fact that MS occurs more frequently in the temperate or northern climates than in tropical areas of the world and more commonly in whites than in blacks. The disease may be acquired in childhood from an outside agent rather than some inherited defect. The natural resistance of the body is important; it is known that certain illnesses and injuries often cause a worsening of the symptoms. Although there are unquestionably mild forms of multiple sclerosis often called benign, many patients ultimately become disabled by symptoms such as weakness and tremor or jerking, with speech becoming less understandable. Urinary and skin problems develop with signs of infection; the patient finally succumbing to some other event apart from actual brain involvement.

Multiple sclerosis is probably the most common non-surgical disease of the nervous system, accounting for the tremendous effort being expended by everyone, and particularly the medical profession, to learn more about this tragic and little understood disease. There are many facts coming to light as the result of research, and the prospects for prevention and treatment will undoubtedly emerge as a result of intensive research into widely different hypotheses or theories of cause and related mechanisms of this illness. Certainly the relationship of slow and persistent viruses is related to many who are suffering from MS or closely related demyelinating diseases.

Evidence also points to the environment that may have an influence exerting its effects in childhood, with a long latent or silent period before disease becomes apparent. Not only is the patient ill but the disease involves his or her family. The patient wishes to be a part of the family as long as possible and close to friends and neighbors. It is estimated that one person out of every thousand will develop MS. The average age of onset of illness is between twenty and forty years with an average length of life of twenty years after onset.

Multiple sclerosis is not only a disease with potentially crippling features, but one producing anxiety, depression and fear as natural consequences of its diagnosis. Dr. B. H. Smith of State University of New York states: "These reactions have inevitable sexual repercussions." Some neurologists advise patients against becoming pregnant. Such warnings may induce a fear of pregnancy reflecting the patient's attitude toward sexual relations.

In 1971 in a review of Multiple Sclerosis, Dr. Uri Leibowitz stated that, "It now seems possible that the central nervous system complications of measles infection may appear in three forms: (1) acute form; (2) subacute form, SSPE; (3) chronic form, MS." "In summary, it would seem that a viral hypothesis can explain most of the epidemiological and experimental data on MS better than any other hypothesis currently available."

┌─ ACKNOWLEDGMENTS ─┐

I WOULD LIKE to express my deep gratitude to the many wonderful people I have known who have MS. I admire their courageous ability to live a restricted life. I thank them, their husbands and/or wives who have taught me a great deal about MS, and to them I dedicate this small book. I wish to express my thanks to several generous donors who have supported my research; and finally to friends and associates who have volunteered many helpful suggestions.

Special recognition and thanks are due my former student Robert A. Good for contributing the Foreword to this book.

J.M.A.

CONTENTS

CONTENTS

MULTIPLE SCLEROSIS
SCARS OF CHILDHOOD
New Horizons and Hope

PART I

─────Chapter 1─────
HISTORICAL NOTES

F RAU ANDRASSY WAS 27, a short sandy-haired woman, mother of two young children. Since the birth of her second child she had lost considerable weight, become anemic, and developed a recurrent throat spasm accompanied by a heaviness in her legs that made it difficult to walk. She was referred to Dr. Sigmund Freud by two doctors who thought the findings indicated neurasthenia without physical causation. Frau Andrassy had been in Dr. Freud's consulting room only a few moments when a foot clonus (a rapid contraction of the muscles) came on. He had her take off her shoe but nothing more. Viennese women had to be examined through their clothing. He massaged her foot until the spasm passed. He then examined her muscular system for symptoms of drawing or pressing, areas of burning, pricking or numbness. He could find none. After he returned to his desk he asked, "these foot spasms apparently do not depress you?" "No, Herr Doktor, I would not compound my difficulties by letting my spirits fall as well." Dr. Freud then said "your condition does not cause you anxiety?" "Not anxiety. I do not have the worrying disposition. Though, naturally we are concerned, my husband and I that it grow no worse. After all I have two small children to raise."

Dr. Freud could find no trace to what to him were the most significant symptoms of neurasthenia: anxiety or a profusion of new maladies, hypochondria. In neurasthenia these were never absent. All the evidence pointed toward an organic disturbance. He must find it.

Dr. Freud turned to his medical bookcase on the wall behind him, and took down one of Charcot's volumes. He read what Dr. Marie said to the group at the Salpetrière: "We can attribute disseminated sclerosis to acute infections incurred in the past." Nothing happened until the patient became undernourished and physically depleted. Under such conditions the weakest point in the spinal cord would revolt; which was exactly what happened to Frau Andrassy. This story is an excerpt from *The Passions of the Mind,* a powerful drama of Sigmund Freud by Irving Stone, and can be dated about 1880 when Dr. Freud was practicing medicine in Vienna. It was in these same years that Jean-Martin Charcot (1825-1893) combined rare talents as a clinician and pathologist. His early work established MS on a firm pathologic basis. Pierre Marie (1853-1940), probably the most eminent of Charcot's students, in a series of lectures on diseases of the spinal cord stated: "*Eruptive Fevers* must also be mentioned, namely, *measles, scarlatina,* and above all *smallpox.* Cases are numerous in which insular [multiple] sclerosis has been known to occur during convalescence after the latter affection: Tremor in the limbs with more or less paresis, disorders of the speech which becomes slow and scanning, nystagmus and in short all the characteristic symptoms of insular sclerosis may exist. At times these symptoms cease and entirely disappear but they may also continue and confirmed insular sclerosis occurs."

Charcot's attention was particularly concerned with attempts to refine and clarify the clinical characteristics of certain neurologic diseases, including MS. He was able to prove that many conditions which were considered diseases were only symptoms. For example, he showed that tremor is not a disease and that there are many kinds of tremor each more or less characteristic of a different disease state. He distinguished the tremor of paralysis agitans and multiple sclerosis which had not been previously separated. If we were to attach a person's name to multiple sclerosis, MS would most certainly have to be called "Charcot's disease."

Toward the end of the 19th century, Devic reported sixteen patients who had visual difficulty known as optic neuritis, associated with involvement of the spinal cord, which caused marked weakness and paralysis of the patient. Early in the twentieth century, patients similar to those originally described by Devic, suffering nearly complete loss of vision with severe involvement of the spinal cord, were reported. In the 1930's Douglas McAlpine and M. Berliner reported several additional patients with Devic's disease. Dr. V. B. Dolgopol (1938) described a case of neuromyelitis optica with pathologic study after death and stated that his patient was unusual because she was a Negro. Devic's syndrome, characterized by severe demyelination, is a subvariety of multiple sclerosis. Dr. F. C. Stansbury recorded the details of five patients with a confirmed diagnosis of neuromyelitis optica and two of his five patients occurred in Negroes, but no particular emphasis was placed on the fact that from a total of twenty cases in his review four were black. A recent review of seventeen black patients studied in a MS clinic revealed that five of seventeen have a confirmed diagnosis of neuromyelitis optica. The most recent edition of *A Textbook of Neurology,* by Dr. H. Houston Merritt states that neuromyelitis optica may occur as the initial symptom of multiple sclerosis or may develop at any time in the course of the disease. The disease may occur at any age, but is more common in children than adults.

On June 27, 1880, Helen Adams Keller was born in Tuscumbia, Alabama. After a normal happy infancy, at about the age of two, she had a severe illness which left her blind and deaf. A recent letter from Alabama Department of Health records a high incidence of measles in 1883. In the winter and spring of 1883, Helen was two years old. Most likely she had measles encephalitis, a rare case of the "scars of childhood."

She grew up and was graduated from Radcliffe College with honors to go on to become one of the world's renowned women until her death in 1968 at the age of eighty-seven.*

---

* A report (1976) from the State of Connecticut Department of Health states that no autopsy was performed on Miss Keller.

Chapter 2
CLINICAL FEATURES
OF MS

By CLINICAL I REFER to how MS affects the patient. Clinically MS may be described as an illness in which the brain and spinal cord are involved by several or many scars which are often quite limited to certain definite areas of the central nervous system, thus accounting for the variability of signs and symptoms. The precise cause of the scars in the brain and spinal cord has not been definitely proved. It is clear that there are many causes but the principal causative factor is related to the common viral infections, many of which occur years before the onset of the signs and symptoms of illness. Childhood infections such as measles, or rubeola, have been most closely implicated with MS. Rarely, other viral infections such as vaccinia (the cowpox virus commonly used to vaccinate against smallpox) are involved. In some individuals viral infections which occur early in life do not disappear after the acute phase but remain hidden or silent only to be activated and reappear in the form of a different illness sometimes in childhood but usually early in adulthood.

The beginning or the first symptoms and signs may follow closely after a stressful experience such as an accident, pregnancy or a new infection. Sometimes stress related to emotional disturbances appears to play a role in the onset of symptoms or such stress may act to aggravate the illness. Overexertion and fatigue occasionally precipitate the first signs, which are blurred vision or weakness and numbness.

The variability of symptoms and signs is related to the various areas of the brain and spinal cord which are involved in the process of forming the scar, "plaque." Scars begin to form around the blood vessels, particularly the veins. Original signs and symptoms of scars in the brain are very minor and cause no concern at once, but in retrospect are frequently recognzed as signs in the early stage of development. Progress of illness is very slow. In many instances the disease continues in a quiescent or benign form. Very careful inquiry into the early signs and symptoms reveals their presence in mild form extending over a considerable period of time dating back even into childhood.

The most typical early symptom relates to visual difficulty or double vision. At times, the nervous system involvement is evidenced by such symptoms as weakness in an arm or a leg, with some difficulty in walking, or numbness and tingling preceding weakness. Weakness or numbness in a single arm or leg is frequently accompanied for a brief period by double vision. Numbness and tingling disappear quickly or in a matter of days and should not be hastily appraised. Neuritis is often sufficient to describe the initial symptoms and signs. Although pain is rarely an early symptom, it is at times attributed to arthritis or a rheumatic symptom. Signs such as numbness and tingling cease and reappear weeks or months after the initial symptoms.

Neuritis involving the visual or optic areas is highly important in arriving at a possible diagnosis of MS. Some blurring in vision occurs temporarily following physical exercise. Testing of vision reveals minor changes in the width of vision with some constriction of the so-called "visual fields." Visual symptoms should be recorded and testing repeated at intervals, as these are among very early signs of illness related to a loss of "myelin," which is the principal defect in MS. A careful examination by the eye specialist reveals some pallor of the optic discs in the back of the eye. This form of multiple sclerosis has been referred to as *neuromyelitis optica*. Visual difficulty occurs as an attack of optic neuritis causing visual loss and some blindness, eventually to be followed by weakness in the legs and definite signs of MS. Occasionally the early symptoms have been diagnosed as acute encephalomyelitis often accompanied by double vision.

The tendency for symptoms and signs to fluctuate is characteristic of MS, and the majority of patients have definite periods when they are free or relieved of symptoms. These periods occasionally last for months or years. In only one patient in every ten do symptoms and signs progress at a steady rate from the beginning. The patient often has true dizziness with loss of balance. Speech is affected and jerkiness or ataxia persists from the beginning. Dr. Douglas McAlpine, recognized as a world authority on multiple sclerosis, followed a large group of patients over a period of ten years. His findings strongly support the concept that a benign form of the disease definitely occurs. An unrestricted course can last for twenty or more years; by contrast, frequent relapses with persisting weakness and ataxia or difficulty with sphincters such as bladder control often point to a more progressive form of the disease. Consequently the process is severe in some body functions whereas it may be very slow or quiescent in others. There is nothing to support the idea that the process is one that is widespread or generalized, involving the whole brain.

Dr. Simon Horenstein, Professor of Neurology, Saint Louis University, wrote recently on "Sexual Dysfunction in Neurological Disease." He states that "with myelopathy associated with multiple sclerosis, the patient retains some perineal muscle control and sensation and often experiences psychogenic erections . . . . Orgasm in the women also follows the same pattern as in men." Professor Horenstein concludes his timely discussion by summarizing his views as follows: "The emotional reaction of the patient including depression or the phobia of the spouse toward the ill person may result in loss of sexual interest or desire though preserved structures and functions make sex feasible.

Chapter 3

ABOUT MEASLES
AND MS

MEASLES IS ONE OF the oldest and most widespread diseases of mankind. The word "measles" could be of German origin: *masa,* meaning the spot. Rubeola and morbilli are other names for measles, but confusing, since in several European countries, rubeola is a word used for rubella or German measles. Rubella and rubeola are two entirely different and distinct diseases caused by their respective viruses.

Historically, measles was undoubtedly recognized by the Arabian physician Rhazes (860-932). A clear description of measles in all of its essential points was made by Thomas Sydenham who reported epidemics in London in 1670 and 1674. He distinguished smallpox, measles and scarlet fever as three separate diseases. Francis Home (1759) produced measles by applying cotton pledges soaked in blood of patients acutely ill with measles to the skin of volunteers. Although measles was suspected of being a virus disease early in the twentieth century, it was not until Doctors John F. Enders and Thomas C. Peebles (1954) were successful in growing the measles virus in tissue culture from throat washings of patients who were early in the eruptive phase of their disease, that the viral cause of measles was proved.

The measles virus is approximately 120 to 220 milli-microns in size, roughly ovoid in shape and contains an inner structure of nucleic acid, surrounded by a protein envelope. Measles virus is included in the subgroup of myxoviruses along with other viruses: Newcastle disease virus, influenza-like viruses and distemper virus in dogs and minks and the virus of a disease in cattle called rinderpest. The measles, distemper and rinderpest viruses are interrelated and may all represent the same virus in their respective hosts: humans, dogs and cattle. A Danish doctor named Ludwig Panum presented the first evidence in 1847 that measles was spread by droplets from the nose and throat sprayed into the air by coughing, one of the classic symptoms of measles.

The definite period of time from the moment of exposure to the first symptoms, called the incubation period, is usually ten to eleven days. The sequence after exposure may be outlined as follows: virus multiplies in the respiratory pas-sages, then spreads to lymph glands and into the blood. Virus continues to multiply in lymph glands until the first symptoms: fever, aching, inflammation about the eyes and conjunctiva, appear. A runny nose and cough result from inflammation in the bronchi of the lungs. Often before the rash develops on the outside of the body, spots appear inside the cheeks. These are known as Koplik's spots, named for the man who first described them. The lining cells of the respiratory passages develop large giant cells first described by Warthin and Finkledey. These cells, so characteristic of measles, are found in almost every organ, including lymph nodes, intestines, tonsils, the appendix and spleen. The disease, then, progresses to the classic eruptive stage appear-ing on the twelfth to fourteenth day after exposure. Rash first appears around the ears but over a period of two to three days it involves the face, spreading downward to involve the trunk, arms and legs. Rash then ceases to be spotty and becomes confluent. Peeling begins in three to four days at which time the rash becomes brownish with some scaling or desquamation. After seven days to two weeks pigmentation and scaling begin to subside and rapid recovery takes place in uncomplicated cases.

A most unusual account of the epidemiology of measles was recorded by Ludwig Panum, a young physician who was sent to the Faroe Islands in 1846 to study an epidemic which occurred there after a measles free interval of sixty-five years. The only previous known epidemic had occurred in 1781. A high percentage of the population of less than 8,000 people was involved; however, over 600 people were ill with measles and 102 deaths resulted.

Panum recorded an incubation period of thirteen to fourteen days and also established the fact that protection was lifelong, as individuals over sixty-five who presumably had had measles in 1781 did not get measles in the widespread epidemic of 1846. Although today we have no specific treatment for measles, a high degree of complacency exists even though this disease may be very serious in some patients. The following quotation is taken from the paper by Panum: "The measles in a disease so generally familiar and so almost trivial that it might be supposed that observations in regard to it could offer nothing new except in special cases with more or less real complications."

Prior to the introduction of the measles vaccine in 1963, over 400 deaths a year from measles occurred in the United States. The death rate has been sharply reduced coincident with the use of the live measles vaccine which causes a mild case of measles sometimes with fever and occasionally with a mild rash, but the patient develops protective antibodies which probably provide lifelong immunity. Very rarely the measles vaccine has resulted in a serious form of encephalitis referred to as subacute sclerosing panencephalitis (SSPE). The incidence following vaccination of this very rare form of measles encephalitis is about the same as that caused by the wild disease prior to the introduction of the vaccine, that is: one per million. Although tragic when it occurs, this event undoubtedly represents a most unusual occurrence and markedly less than the overall protection enjoyed by the children who are successfully vaccinated against measles. The measles virus may persist in the body and account for lifetime immunity enjoyed by the majority of human beings who have recovered from measles.

The long-range consequences of aftereffects of the live measles vaccine are still unknown, because insufficient time has elapsed to assess its full effect. SSPE may occur five to twenty years after childhood measles, and the interval may be much longer in the more chronic aftereffect such as MS.

The complications of measles are severe, one severe form consists of bleeding, which on occasion has been referred to as "black measles." Another very serious complication is measles encephalitis, which may occur at any time during the course of the disease. Most recently this serious complication has been considered to be caused by the measles virus. However, the isolation of the virus directly from the brain and spinal fluid has been difficult but has now been accomplished in several laboratories. The most important evidence that the measles virus is primarily responsible for the changes in measles encephalitis resulted from the finding that fatal cases of measles encephalitis show all the classical findings produced by the measles virus in the body; these consist primarily of virus inclusion bodies found in the brain cells in experimental as well as natural measles. When studied by the light and electron microscope, the changes are identical with those known to be caused by proved measles infection in tissue culture cells.

The symptoms of measles encephalitis may begin either abruptly or gradually and vary from a mild delirium, a convulsion or a deep coma. The earliest symptoms are restlessness, headache, vomiting and convulsions which occur in about one half of all patients. The electro-encephalogram (EEG) is abnormal and the spinal fluid shows an increase in white blood cells and an elevation of protein. Although measles is a worldwide disease and probably occurs in almost 100 percent of the exposed population, the true incidence of measles might be approximately equal to the birth rate. In England the measles known verification rate is only about 60 percent of the birth rate. Varying rates of encephalitis have been reported but the most widely accepted rate is about one per 1,000 reported cases of measles.

To summarize, common measles (rubeola) is an extremely important worldwide disease. The measles virus could be classified as one of the common cold viruses characterized by cough, coryza (a runny nose), conjunctivitis and a blotchy red rash. Measles virus may cause serious disease without a rash. The most important consequence of measles is measles encephalitis, occurring in about one in 1,000 cases. A safe and effective vaccine for the prevention of measles is available and should be given to everyone who has not had the regular measles. German measles (rubella) is an entirely different disease and is serious for the unborn baby when it attacks the mother early in pregnancy. The rubella virus may rarely cause encephalitis but does not cause serious demyelinating disease which is so characteristic of MS, now clearly related to the rubeola or measles virus, and other virus-like agents.

Chapter 4

MILD OR BENIGN MS

Ms has a bad reputation. Although the reputation of a severe illness is justified in some cases, strong evidence suggests that on occasion MS is a mild disorder indeed. It may be mild at the beginning, during the development of the illness, or ultimately may remain silent for years or forever. Difficulty in categorizing the degree of severity is due to the widely varied manifestations of the illness. Because of unusual clinical findings or lack of any clear symptoms or signs, the labels "probable" or "possible" MS are the first terms used until symptoms or signs become more extensive. Changes in the eyes such as pallor of the discs may suggest possible MS. A definite diagnosis of MS particularly in the early stages of illness is unlikely, lacking a specific diagnostic test. Elevated antibodies to certain viruses in blood serum or spinal fluid lead the doctor to strongly suspect that a "slow-virus" may be active in the patient's body, causing symptoms of MS even though they are very mild.

Many years ago Doctor Douglas McAlpine published the results of a study of 241 patients he followed closely for ten or more years. He formulated a classification according to the degree of disability. In MS the major cause of disability comes from the weakness in one or both lower limbs or a lack of balance or a combination of these symptoms.

He developed a type of yardstick or measure of a patient's abilities. First, he spoke of "Unrestricted" which he defined as without restriction of activity for normal employment or domestic purposes but not necessarily symptom free. A second category he called "Restricted" and defined this group as those who are able to walk unaided for short distances up to half a mile and able to get on and off public transport. A third group he called "Markedly Restricted" and defined these patients as capable of moving outdoors without difficulty for up to a quarter of a mile usually with the aid of sticks, and often unable to use public transport. The fourth group was called "Mobility-at-Home," and here the patient is able to move with difficulty about the house with support from furniture but unable to mount stairs. The fifth category is "Immobility-at-Home" confined to chair or wheelchair and entirely dependent on others for moving from room to room. The final group he states are "Bedridden." Results of his long study of 241 patients are as follow: dead 83; disabled 80; and 78 were unrestricted. The degree of disability in the eighty disabled group showed that of those followed for fifteen to twenty years a significant proportion were not severely incapacitated. One third of the whole series or seventy-eight patients at the end of the ten-year period were without restriction for normal employment or domestic life but were not necessarily symptom free. An acute form may affect the vision partially, and if in certain patients the symptoms remain mild after ten years the outlook is quite favorable.

Other reports in medical literature on mild forms of MS state that any case may be considered mild if it permits a more or less normal social and occupational career after a long course under partial remission. A report from St. Joseph's Hospital in Paris records 300 patients studied who had MS for ten and fifteen years. The disease was present for fifteen years in thirty-three of their patients; in eighteen the course of the disease was mild for ten years and found still to be so after fifteen. A mild form of disease had persisted in two patients for thirty-one and thirty-seven years respectively. They conclude that the benign forms of MS present from the early stages of the disease allow hope of a favorable outlook in 20 percent of all cases. Another report of interest recorded two "clinically silent" patients discovered to have MS only at autopsy. In summary the authors state that the uniformly evil reputation of MS justified in some cases is certainly not justified in others. The neurologist sees a biased selection of the "worst" cases and does not see many in whom the disease is less severe. A study of 900 relatives of MS patients reported twenty-one definite and seven possible cases of the disease. In another report sixty-six cases of MS were found among 15,644 autopsies. Twelve or 18 percent had not been clinically suspected. The authors believe that one silent MS case occurs in each four definitely diagnosed.

Recognition of the "benign" form of MS leads to three possible conclusions. *First,* the gloomy outlook cast by the diagnosis must certainly be modified. *Second,* a more positive attitude should be taken toward the question of treatment. *Third,* in a certain proportion of patients where resistance is high it seems possible that a more prolonged period of rest and aftercare in the early stages of the disease might beneficially influence the subsequent course of the disease. Pierre Marie (1895) in discussing the course of MS referred to a type with permanent improvement or even recovery and the possibility of arrest during any part of the course. Other quotations from the world literature provide hope for patients with multiple sclerosis. "It is probable that in a few rare and exceptional cases the disease is permanently arrested" . . . "Patients in whom the initial disturbance is relatively sudden may remain in perfect health for months or years at a time." Lord Brain, one of the world's most distinguished neurologists, summarized his views on the outlook for MS when he wrote: "If a remission may last thirty years, why not for a lifetime?"

Two patients seen by the author recently were sixty-one and sixty-five years of age, having had MS for 36 and 38 years respectively—striking reminders of the benign form of MS.

PART II

PART II

—Chapter 5—
DISTRIBUTION OF MS
IN THE WORLD

THE NEUROLOGIST AND researcher interested in the "why of MS" studies the distribution of MS in the world in search of clues to the possible cause. Over the years the findings show that although MS is worldwide in distribution there are regions where the disease is more common than elsewhere. High and low frequency areas correspond to the cold and hot regions of the world being highest in the colder and lowest in the warmer regions. The high risk areas are in the temperate zones whereas the low risk areas are near the tropics in both northern and southern hemispheres.

Two viral diseases which are also worldwide share a parallelism with MS; they are regular measles (rubeola) and poliomyelitis. The first epidemic of poliomyelitis was recognized in northern Sweden about 1840. In the United States the first polio epidemic occurred in Vermont in 1910. Paralytic polio or "infantile paralysis" as it was originally diagnosed is rare in tropical regions of the world. The viruses of poliomyelitis are present in the tropics; but the paralytic forms of the disease are very uncommon. Measles is worldwide and like MS and polio is recognized as involving the nervous system more commonly in the colder regions of the world such as the Faroe Islands, north of Scotland, where severe epidemics occurred. Measles encephalitis, the most serious form of the disease, is rare in Africa and tropical climates. The parallelism is obvious.

The best way to identify a viral disease is by the specific antibodies it produces. When patients with MS were compared with persons who did not have MS, Doctor J. K. Clarke and associates (1965) found that antibodies in the blood were higher in the MS patients against measles virus, but not against the polio viruses.

That high and low risk areas for MS do exist in the world is a well-established fact, but the precise reason for the discrete differences is not known. A hypothesis regarding the significance of hygiene and sanitation has been suggested with scant data to support the concept. In the developing countries where hygiene is frequently poor the risk of developing MS is low. On the contrary, where the level of hygiene and sanitation is good, the prevalence of MS is at medium or high incidence. In the low hygiene regions, the newborn may receive a high degree of protection from his mother, and in the early years may acquire natural active immunity in a safe manner from the environment. The individual grows up with a substantial degree of protection against common infectious diseases such as measles and poliomyelitis. When confronted by an epidemic or exposure, the illness may be mild or inapparent, bolstering his immunity to even higher levels.

The child who approaches childhood and school in the high hygiene environment is the one who may be the sickest with viremia and at a higher risk of developing aftereffects. Doctor Uri Leibowitz and associates (1966) reported that the level of hygiene and sanitation did make a significant difference, patients with disease reported higher standards of sanitation than control persons with low levels of hygiene.

A recent question proposed by Dr. Milton Alter (1976)

asks: "Is MS an age-dependent response to measles?" In the tropics, MS is rare and children tend to acquire measles before age three. In temperate areas, measles tends to be acquired later after age five. Alter states that "If MS is a response of the patient to having measles later in childhood, then, mass measles vaccination programs should produce a decline in the rate of MS."

Epidemiologists have chosen to divide the world into three frequency zones for MS. They define a high zone or high prevalence at 30 to 60 per 100,000 population. A medium zone ranges from 5 to 15 and the low prevalence at less than 5 per 100,000 population. Most reports by the epidemiologists show a division of multiple sclerosis frequency into high-medium-low divisions. The high risk areas consist of northern Europe and northern United States, much of southern Canada, New Zealand and probably southern Australia. Epidemiologists speak of prevalence rates in the areas just referred to as averaging 30 to 80 per 100,000, centering about 50. Frequency in the middle zones averages 10 to 15 per 100,000. In Europe, the Mediterranean area is considered medium with a dividing line across France and southern Switzerland. Romania is considered in the middle with respect to the prevalence of MS, and Turkey measures low. The west coast of Norway and all Scandinavia above latitude 65°N are also in the middle area of frequency.

In regard to the USSR the northwest area is high, central and southern medium, similar to southern United States and most of Australia. Practically all sites in Asia, the Pacific Islands, Africa, Latin America, Alaska and Greenland are low risk. The prevalence rate may be defined as the number of cases present in a given community at one time divided by the population of the community at the same time. So the rate may be expressed as a ratio of cases over the population. For example: in a small town with a population of 350 people where seven persons have MS, the prevalence rate is seven per 350. We are looking for clues to the cause of multiple sclerosis by further detailed studies in high risk areas.

A recent study by Koch and associates (1974) described a concentration of cases of MS in a small town in the state of Washington. They reported six patients who were born in the small community all of whom had a diagnosis of MS verified by physicians and reaffirmed by specialists in neurology. Such a concentration referred to as a "cluster" would give a spurious high prevalence rate. The diagnosis of MS always is a risk as in many instances the diagnosis can only be confirmed by autopsy.

As pointed out by Dr. John F. Kurtzke (1975), there is very little reason to correlate the distribution of multiple sclerosis with the latitude of the area, and to be meaningful, longitude must also be considered. He states, for example, that latitude 40°N is a high frequency zone in America, medium in Europe and low in Asia. In the northern hemisphere all the high and medium prevalence regions are in Europe or in places colonized by Europeans. It seems likely that MS originated in western Europe and spread from there to the United States and Canada as well as to New Zealand and Australia.

In order to evaluate distribution throughout the world, reported studies require a critical review of their comparability. Since we are dealing with a rare disease and the diagnosis is always at risk, especially in benign cases when diagnosis can only be confirmed at atopsy, meaningful prevalence rates are certainly subject to error. Kurtzke concludes "there will probably be no perfect study on the frequency of MS. It is a fact that all the high risk and medium risk areas are found in Europe or in regions colonized by Europeans."

In Korea the prevalence rate of MS has been estimated

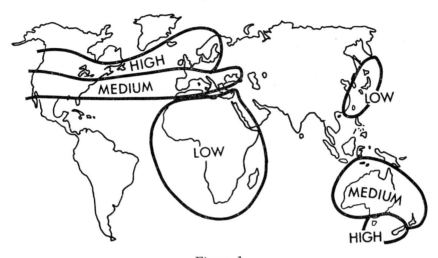

Figure 1.
From J. H. D. Millar, *Multiple Sclerosis.* Springfield, Thomas, 1971.
Courtesy of Charles C Thomas, Publisher.

to be 2/100,000. Similar estimates exist for India and Japan. Neuromyelitis optica, a form of MS, is frequently diagnosed in Korea and Japan, possibly accounting for the low prevalence rate of MS. A typical case was reported from Seoul National University in a six-year-old boy who was admitted to the hospital because of a sudden loss of visual acuity and paralysis of legs of seven days' duration. He improved in two weeks, but finally remained unchanged for five months. His doctors diagnosed the illness as neuromyelitis optica, not MS.

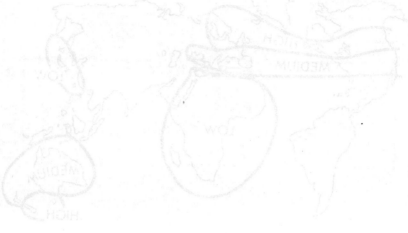

Chapter 6

DEMYELINATION AND RELATED DISEASES

PATHOLOGY OF MS

Myelin is the material which surrounds the nerves in the brain. Since its injury and destruction is the primary change which occurs in multiple sclerosis, what does demyelination in the nervous system really mean? The destruction or disappearance of myelin sheaths from the nerve tracts may be due to injury or disease of the blood vessels related to lack of proper nutrition, or an infectious process. We can speak of primary demyelinating diseases, or when the casual agent is unknown demyelination might be secondary to hereditary or other causes. It is important to attempt to arrange demyelinating processes in relation to *time* as acute or subacute forms and finally, chronic manifestations. It is likewise difficult to arrange demyelinating diseases on the basis of the injury or pathologic change seen in the brain. An attempt to arrange or classify these illnesses on the basis of the symptoms and signs that the patient shows also is difficult if not impossible.

In his textbook on *Diseases of the Nervous System*, Lord Brain (1962) arranged the demyelinating disorders first as acute encephalomyelitis following acute infections such as

31

measles, chicken pox, smallpox, vaccination against smallpox and rabies. In a further subdivision he speaks of disseminated or multiple myelitis associated with optic neuritis. A third variety and one which is of primary concern in this chapter is disseminated or multiple sclerosis.

These subdivisions as designated by Lord Brain will be discussed in the following sections. First, acute disseminated encephalomyelitis is characterized by a loss of, or injury to, myelin about blood vessels in the brain and spinal cord. It is usually related to virus diseases such as measles, rubella, smallpox, mumps, chicken pox, and vaccination against smallpox. Injury to myelin may occur spontaneously. In other words, no obvious cause is apparent. The tissue changes in the brain and spinal cord are centered about the veins, and many cells such as lymphocytes or plasma cells gather about the space around the veins. The changes occur mostly in the white matter of the brain where the nerve tracts gather together and are covered with myelin. These changes are rarely seen in the outer part or gray matter of the brain. Changes are referred to as inflammatory and occur throughout the nervous system. It is possible that the inflammatory and early destructive changes about the veins cease and result in partial or complete recovery. The many different viruses which cause encephalitis produce almost identical changes but vary in severity depending on factors such as heredity, age, and the character of the causal agent; some produce much more severe changes than others. Rubeola or measles virus is one of the most devastating viruses which attacks the nervous system. Some viruses produce inflammation in the brain with very little demyelination. The mechanism of injury is not always clear. The rubella virus causes encephalitis but minimal evidence of demyelination. It is not related to MS.

Encephalomyelitis following vaccination against smallpox is a rare complication. It occurs more commonly following the first vaccination rather than at the time of revaccination. Symptoms of encephalomyelitis following vaccination usually occur about the tenth to twelfth day although nervous symptoms have been reported on the second day and as late as the twenty-fifth day. The first symptoms are headache, drowsiness, vomiting, and fever, and occasionally convulsions. Diagnosis of vaccination encephalitis is not difficult because the patient has had a recent vaccination, signs of which may still be seen. Otherwise, it may be difficult to distinguish vaccination encephalitis from other forms of acute encephalomyelitis, particularly those complicating rash diseases such as measles and chicken pox.

The occurrence of encephalitis in association with smallpox has been known for many years but considered to be a rare complication occurring in only one or two patients per thousand suffering from smallpox. The changes in the nervous system are similar to those that occur following vaccination against smallpox.

Encephalomyelitis complicating measles is essentially the same as a complication of smallpox vaccination. Research studies reported by the author in 1966 and subsequent reports have clearly implicated the measles virus as the cause of the injury and destructive changes in the brain. It was not until 1954 that J. F. Enders and T. C. Peebles isolated measles virus in tissue culture and thus established the injuring effects caused by the virus. Cells become fused together and are referred to as a giant cell. Virus inclusion bodies occur in infected cells. When these are studied by the electron microscope, dense and fuzzy tubules are seen in cells proved to be infected by measles virus. The changes are intimately related to viral inclusion bodies seen with the light microscope occurring in the inflamed tissues particularly about the blood vessels in the brain and spinal cord.

The most recent report of measles encephalitis was made

by V. ter Meulen and associates in December 1972. An
intensive and detailed study was made of a forty-year-old
man who developed encephalitis three days after the onset
of measles. The patient died six weeks later and the autopsy
showed changes which were consistent with measles
encephalitis. Fresh brain tissue from the patient was inoculated into tissue cultures and when cultivated directly or
in conjunction with cells from a monkey the measles virus
was identified. Pictures in their article showed a large area
of demyelination referred to as "plaque." An area of inflammation was also shown as well as viral inclusion bodies in
the cytoplasm and nucleus of the cells. The final conclusion
by ter Meulen and his associates following the successful
isolation of the measles virus was that their patient died
from measles encephalitis, caused by the measles virus. The
changes seen in the microscope were similar to the late
scarring type known to be associated with measles encephalitis and MS. This patient represents a case of acute, subacute or chronic demyelinating disease proved to be caused
by the measles virus.

Old Dog Encephalitis (ODE) provides a model for
further study of the cause and pathogenesis of severe demyelinating diseases in man. This disease occurs in *mature* dogs
that develop a chronic form of encephalitis, with difficulty
in walking (ataxia), rare convulsions, and circling.

Pathologic findings in mature dogs with ODE are compared with the findings in MS, SSPE and NO (neuromyelitis
optica) in man. Optic neuritis in dogs with chronic distemper shows changes similar to those in the optic tract
of human patients with severe demyelinating disease. The
pathologic changes in MS, such as perivascular infiltration
with lymphocytes, plasma cells and demyelination are similar
to those seen in ODE. The findings strongly support a
possible relationship of ODE to multiple sclerosis, subacute
sclerosing panencephalitis, and neuromyelitis optica.

The classic pathologic features of a typical case of MS, according to Dr. C. E. Lumsden (1970), are so striking that no disease has more characteristic findings than the pattern of changes observed in the central nervous system. The pattern is a combination of many kinds of alterations of the brain and the extent of the involvement is often small when the disability of the particular patient is considered. Some of the scarred areas in the brain appear to be old whereas others are small and appear to be quite new. They are so different from the old areas of scarring as to be easily missed. Areas of the involvement are randomly scattered throughout the central nervous system. As originally pointed out by Charcot, in the most severe cases, no area of the brain is spared. Lumsden points out that there is no question that MS is a demyelinating process and myelin covering the nerve tracks represents the prime target at risk. In the majority of cases the area about the veins is involved and these may join together and form what might be considered a patch of myelin destruction or a *scar* rarely bigger than a small coin or about one inch in diameter. 2037546

The appearance of the patches seen at postmortem are so characteristic and striking that the skilled pathologist has no difficulty in recognizing them as the scars of MS.

In two separate research studies antibodies in the spinal fluid against the vaccinia virus have been found in about 30 percent of patients with MS. The vaccinia virus was implicated in the death of a thirteen-year-old girl who was vaccinated at the age of seven months. She was quite well until the age of eleven when she had visual difficulty which was diagnosed as optic neuritis and this was followed by paralysis in her legs. After her death, brain material was inoculated into rabbits; all developed vaccinia antibodies. None of the uninoculated rabbits in the same room developed vaccinia antibodies. Brain studies showed the changes which are known to be caused by the vaccinia virus. This case implicated the vaccinia virus as the cause of neuromyelitis optica or Devic's disease. This disease occurs more commonly in children than in adults, but it may occur rarely from five to sixty years of age. The spinal cord may be involved very early even before the brain with the possible exception of the optic nerve which is an important part of the brain. The experienced pathologist states that there is no doubt about the fact that the earliest areas of involvement are those around the veins. The optic nerve or the main nerve of the eye is highly vulnerable in this disease.

It should be pointed out that the majority of patients with multiple sclerosis die from diseases other than the primary involvement of the brain and spinal cord. It is true that a high incidence of malnutrition and chronic infection may occur in patients with MS, but no consistent disease association has been observed. Almost without exception the optic pathways to the brain from the eye are involved in MS. From this discussion the *cause* of multiple sclerosis cannot be determined by the pathologic changes found in the classic cases. However, pathology is the indispensable compass by which the current experimental and epidemiological research must be steered and without which research may be meaningless.

Chapter 7

PREVENTION AND TREATMENT

IMMUNOLOGY

P REVENTION AND TREATMENT of disease depend not only on how we protect ourselves from, but also on how we defend ourselves against invaders such as viruses. Some viruses persist in the body of the infected person for months or years, even though antibodies against the particular virus are also present. There are several well-known examples of persistent viral infections in man. One is the virus of the common cold sore, the herpes simplex virus (HSV). A closely related virus to herpes is called cytomegalovirus (or "big cell"), because the virus produces a large body in the infected cells called an inclusion body. These viral inclusion bodies occur in herpes and in certain cells when infected by the regular measles virus, rubeola.

Slow or persistent viruses were first discovered in animals with a neurological disease which the veterinarians called *scrapie*. This disease in sheep got its name because the animals rubbed themselves against fence posts. The illness which caused the itching eventually caused a stumbling gait and weakness of the legs, and finally, collapse. This disease in sheep had a very long incubation period. As long as three to five years might elapse following contact with other infected animals before the onset of symptoms. The sheep finally ended up with disease of the brain. This disease in sheep differs in many respects from slow virus diseases in human beings.

A disease of human beings now considered a slow virus disease was discovered among cannibalistic Stone Age man in the high interior of New Guinea. This disease is called *kuru,* which stands for shivering. These people have a marked tremor and shivering-like symptoms even though they live in a tropical climate. Infected individuals have difficulty in walking and a slurring of speech which eventually results in their inability to talk. They also have jerky eye movements, but no true nystagmus, which is one of the classic symptoms of MS. Mentality remains quite normal even though the disease, once it has developed, progresses to a fatal outcome. Patients with *kuru* do not have the typical demyelination so characteristic of MS; but they do have a type of inflammation in the brain which is characterized by increased numbers of cells called astrocytes This disease was common in children and their mothers who often remained at home while the father was away hunting. The women and children who remained home indulged in cannibalism. The brains of the people they ate were considered a delicacy. Many of the people who were cannibalized had *kuru.* Now that cannibalism has been stopped, the disease has become very rare, and at last count no children under fourteen were known to have *kuru.*

A definition of a slow virus infection was first provided by B. Sigurdsson, an Icelandic veterinarian, who described an infection in sheep caused by an agent which produced a progressive disease lasting over a period of months and years with a long incubation period, leading to an infection in a particular or single organ such as the brain.

The immune systems of the body are responsible for checking the destructive ability of viruses, and on occasion may even be responsible for some of the manifestations of an infection. The way the immune system stops viral infections is related to the way the virus spreads in the body. A virus spreads from one cell to another when cells are multiplying or dividing. The first type of spread is usually stopped by antibodies in the blood called "humoral" antibodies. These antibodies attach themselves to the viruses and destroy them. This attachment forms what the immunologists now call a virus-antibody complex. Humoral antibody neutralizes the virus by covering the surface and thus preventing its attachment to cells. The straightforward neutralization of virus particles sometimes occurs with the aid of a substance called complement.

Another mechanism of cellular immunity consists of inflammatory cells such as lymphocytes and plasma cells which prevent viruses from fusing, thus interfering with their spread.

Certain immune lymphocytes exude a toxin called lymphotoxin and also interferon (see Chapter 9), a protein substance which prevents a virus from multiplying and thus prevents other cells from becoming infected. Interferon may protect a very large number of cells in a certain organ such as the liver or the brain. Certain cells in the body make interferon much better than other cells and agents such as viruses or bacteria stimulate or induce the production of interferon by cells. The mechanism is called "cell-mediated" immune response.

It is still an unanswered question as to why in the presence of the various immune systems of the body, viruses can remain hidden, persisting in certain cells and continuing to damage them. In some instances viruses infect the cells of the immune system, such as in leukemia, and thus depress the immune response of the individual. This depression of the immune response is referred to as binding or interfering with antiviral antibody.

The next important questions to be answered are: (1) can effective means such as vaccines be developed to prevent or to control persistent infections, and (2) is there any way to cure persons once they become chronically infected? Certainly one approach to prevention is to induce or encourage the production of interferon. A second possibility is to stimulate the immune responses of the body to combat infection. The cells in the immune system of the body begin their development in the liver during the life of the baby before birth. These basic cells then operate through the thymus gland to produce certain types of lymphocytes known as T-cells and some of them operate through the bone marrow and produce another type of immune cell known as the "B" lymphocyte. This B cell may become a plasma cell which lives only a day or two but plays a very important role in the immune systems of the body making it possible for us to defend ourselves against invading viruses which aids in the cause of the disease.

The antibodies formed in the body do not help us recover from an infection, but they do prevent getting the disease a second or third time. The main role of the immune system is prevention. The cells which develop from the thymus and bone marrow play a very important role in combating infection and ridding the body of certain infections. When the body lacks the ability to defend itself, rare deficiency diseases result because the body lacks immune antibodies and immune cells which are needed to keep us well. When we are deficient in certain immune mechanisms we suffer from infectious diseases, and these can be fatal in the individual who lacks the ability of defense through the immune systems.

We must think of treatment in terms of prevention.

Smallpox, poliomyelitis and measles can be prevented by inoculation of a safe and modified form of the virus, inducing the production of antibodies which do not cure disease but prevent infection by the specific infecting agent or virus. Although the possibility of treatment of MS by encouraging and stimulating the immune mechanisms is under intensive study and research the best *treatment* at present is *prevention*. The fact that many patients with MS related to viral infections which have become chronic or persistent have periods of feeling better and of actually improving to the point of partial recovery if not complete suggests that direct treatment is a reality. This event is referred to as a remission or a ceasing of the symptoms and these periods may last for months and even years. They lend hope to the fact that immune systems can be encouraged and induced to produce a period of recovery or a remission This is the direct attack against chronic viral infections. Doctor Lynn E. Spitler reports: "Research which can stimulate immune responses is at the threshold of medical practice."

One of the first agents to be discovered and developed is *transfer factor* (TR). To create TR a donor must be found whose blood has a natural immune response to the subject's disease. The acceptable donor will spend approximately four hours while all the blood in his body is processed to "separate out" TR. is blood flows into a cell separator, a centrifuge device where the red blood cells settle to the bottom, the plasma rises to the top, and the white blood cells stay near the center. The white cells are siphoned out and frozen, turning them into a white powder. This powder, containing TR, can be injected into the patient suffering with the specific disease or infection to increase resistance to the illness.

Patients with MS may have a viral infection affecting the brain, since these patients have a measured difference in their immune response to measles leading researchers to suspect that MS may be an ongoing measles virus infection. This suggests therapy using immune response agents, i.e. TR.

BCG (Bacillus Calmette-Gerin) is a bacterial substance considered to increase cellular immunity. However, it may also cause undesirable side effects. Another chemical substance that stimulates cellular immunity without serious side effects is an agent called levamisole. This drug boosts cellular immunity particularly if cell-mediated immunity is depressed. Spitler found that levamisole helped to control recurrent infections with herpes viruses. It is truly an antiviral agent.

Reports in the medical literature record favorable results from the use of levamisole in Herpes virus infections, influenza and hepatitis. Owners of animals with ODE report improvement or remission in their dogs to us.[*]

Levamisole restores immune functions particularly in cells involved in cell-mediated immune reactions. Levamisole has been used successfully is several diseases of man, including recurrent and chronic infections.

[*] Harold Snow, D.V.M. and the author.

Chapter 8

RECENT RESEARCH ON
MULTIPLE SCLEROSIS

P ERSPECTIVES IN MULTIPLE SCLEROSIS" was the subject of a two-day program sponsored by the National Institute of Neurological and Communciative Disorders and Stroke held at the National Institutes of Health, Bethesda, Maryland, early in 1975. At this conference, research investigators from all over the world gathered to exchange new information they had gained from researches about MS. One of the most interesting aspects of the conference was the emphasis on the patient (host)—why some develop disease while others do not.

In a paper concerned with genetic factors in multiple sclerosis, several diseases were discussed but only in MS was a strong association of lymphocyte determinants observed. The authors reported that in patients with MS an increased frequency of HL-A3 and HL-A7 types was observed, confirming findings previously observed is several other laboratories.

The influence of the genetic factors on the clinical course of the disease had been analyzed, and only among patients who carry the HL-A7 or the LD-7a genetic determinant was rapidly developing disease observed. These investigators found an association between the occurrence of high measles

43

antibodies in MS patients who carry HL-A3, 7 and/or W18 suggesting that genetic factors contribute to the control of antibody production. No conclusion was reached as little is known about the component of the measles virus involved in this activity. These authors did state that the leukocyte migration test (MIF) was the rationale behind the treatment of MS patients with Transfer Factor (TR) the substance which normalizes the reactivity. Finally, it was evident from their studies that the LD-7a is a genetic determinant which occurs in 60 to 70 percent of patients with MS, and this when compared to 16 percent in normal unrelated individuals provides some insight into genetic factors in MS.

A second group of investigators reported immunologic factors as they relate to the genetics of demyelinating disease. The authors agreed with the previously outlined report that HL-A3 and HL-A7 types are over-represented in MS when compared to control populations, and they also agreed that LD-7a is strikingly over-represented in MS. Measles antibodies tend to be higher in MS patients than in controls, but persons who bear HL-A3 have higher measles antibody titers than those who do not, whether or not they have MS. Measles antibody titers were higher in the serum of patients with MS than in those individuals with LD-7a, and also higher in brothers and sisters.

A third report analyzed HL-A in nine families in which at least two individuals had MS. This brief preliminary report was inconclusive, but it suggested that differences in exposure to environmental factors such as measles virus may explain why not all individuals with the genetic susceptibility develop the disease. It is possible that immune deficiency is why some individuals are more susceptible than others to common childhood illnesses. Also the occurrence of measles late in childhood might increase the likelihood of acquiring MS.

The difficulties of evaluating any form of treatment were emphasized. A theoretical basis for attacking the genetic relationship in MS was cited since HL-A studies have shown a dominance of the 7a type and its correlation with progression of disease.

Another report concerned immunologic studies with TR in MS. Several investigators were involved in this study which was headed by Dr. John B. Zabriskie. They found a selective cellular suppression to measles virus was present in patients with MS. It was this selective suppression which prompted the investigation of TR and the ability of cells in the body and in the test tube to react to measles virus. The authors selected individuals who exhibited a high degree of reactivity to measles virus and these individuals provided the TR used in their study. Fifteen patients were studied and eleven developed significantly higher values to measles virus following the use of TR. The majority of their patients exhibited an increased response to measles virus. Increased migration values continued for six weeks following the injection of TR.

The last paper in this series was a further study of immunity in patients with MS. Serum from patients with MS inhibited the immune release in lymphocytes from patients with measles-infected cells. These data suggest the lymphocyte "killer" function in patients with MS.

A recently published report on *visna,* a chronic inflammatory demyelinating disease in the central nervous system of sheep, throws further light on the problem of how a virus is able to persist in the host and become a "slow virus." Sheep provide an animal model to study the phenomenon of persistence, thus having potential application in the study of MS. The visna virus produces a severe crippling demyelinating disease in sheep; however, there is no evidence that it has any counterpart disease in human beings.

Another recently published report by Dr. Richard I.

Carp and associates showed that mouse tissue culture cells were markedly inhibited in their growth when exposed to brain and spleen tissues from patients with MS. Originally these researchers tested samples from ten cases of MS and found a reduction in the total cells in their cultures treated with brain material from MS patients. They then tested samples from seventy-one MS patients and samples from forty-five non-MS patients. These cultures showed a reduction in the yield from the MS material when compared to control non-MS) material. The presence of the agent responsible for the decrease was not limited to the brain and spleen tissue from patients but was also found in the serum and cerebrospinal fluid and in kidney tissue and lymph nodes from MS patients. It was concluded that the cause of the reduction in the cell yields was high in the mice treated with MS material, but no response was observed in samples from the non-MS patients.

The virus-like agent found in association with MS patients initially delineated by Carp and associates is small and similar in size to the scrapie agent, discussed previously in Chapter 7. The changes caused by the Carp agent are also produced by the scrapie agent. An important difference between the agents is that the effect produced by the Carp agent can be neutralized by sera from MS patients; no such neutralization has been detected in scrapie. This research represents an important milestone in MS and offers hope in the search for new answers.*

A report on the relationship between measles virus antibodies and oligoclonal immune globulin (IgG) in cerebrospinal fluid (CSF) in patients with MS was presented by Doctors Erling Norrby and Bodvar Vandik, from the Karolinska Institutet, Stockholm, Sweden. Measles virus antibody occurred in the serum and C.S.F. of 80 percent

---

* THE LANCET, February 28, 1976.

of patients with MS. Several methods to study measles antibodies in the serum and spinal fluid were used to compare patients with MS and with SSPE. These authors concluded that in the patient with SSPE the IgG represents an oligoclonal IgG response to a high level of antibody against the measles virus.

Studies with the electron microscope were presented with pictures of tissue culture cells infected with the SSPE virus and measles virus. Brain material from patients dying with MS were studied with the electron microscope and changes were similar to those initially reported in 1972 by John W. Prineas. The structural changes were much like those found previously in association with cells proved to be infected with the measles virus. Figure 2 shows the measles virus magnified thousands of times; the picture is similar to the changes observed in the brain of patients with SSPE and MS.

Figure 2 appears on the following page.

←—————————— Figure 2.

Figure 2.   Intertwined tubules fill the nucleus of a cell. These fine threads are measles virus particles magnified 61,000 times with the electron microscope. The picture was taken by W. Jann Brown from a specimen kindly provided by L. S. Oshira, of the California State Department of Public Health.

─────Chapter 9─────
INTERFERON – An Antiviral

INTERFERON, DISCOVERED IN 1957 by Alick Isaacs and Jean Lindenmann (although slowly accepted by the practicing physician), has proved to be a defense mechanism in recovery from acute and sometimes chronic infections. It is a most important component of the body's defenses against many different kinds of infections and particularly viral infections. As one of the body's first defenses against invading organisms, it acts sooner than the humoral and cell-mediated antibodies. In fact, interferon is the major determinant in recovery from illness by inducing the formation of a substance in body cells which interfere with the multiplication of viruses. It not only arrests the multiplication and spread of viruses but also is active in actual destruction of viruses and prevention of reinfection. Interferon's importance extends beyond its action against viruses; in fact, it has been shown to have an antagonistic effect against bacteria, rickettsia and protozoa. The name implies an interference with processes of development of cancer where the effects of interferon are also under intensive investigation.

Interferon is not in itself directly antiviral but induces the formation of a new substance which activates the antiviral mechanism. There are at least two ways in which interferon acts with cells to produce the antiviral effect. First, it stimulates the production of another substance by cells, which is directly antiviral. Or, a small amount of interferon works in combination with cell components to produce an antiviral state. Antibodies on the other hand inhibit viral infections by combining with the virus and making it noninfectious for cells. Antibodies are usually produced after infection, serving mainly to prevent reinfection and to promote resistance to reinfection. The effective role of existing antibody is primarily one of prevention and it is questionable whether antibody is effective after the viral infection has become established in the body. Most of the experimental evidence supports a direct relationship between the interferon system and recovery from infections.

The control of virus diseases may be approached from several points of view. First, immunologic control is accomplished by prevention through the development of vaccines. A second approach to control is through certain chemical substances which have antiviral activity. An example is a chemical known as iododeoxyuridine (IDU) which has been shown to have an antiviral effect against Herpes viruses types one and two. The third approach to control is to heighten resistance of the host (the patient) exemplified by the interferon mechanism. Living cells in the body infected by viruses produce interferon, a process independent of antibody formation. Interferon's early antiviral activity has a protective effect evident before the presence of antibodies' can be demonstrated. Interferon can be found in body fluids, in the blood and spinal fluid in patients early in the course of their disease. An example is influenza where it is found in the fluids from the nose, and in influenza meningitis in spinal fluid. In summary, interferon provides the first line of defense against infection, acting on the cells and preventing further spread of infection. As stated previously the main function of antibody is to prevent reinfection. The fate of the individual cell depends on substances other than antibody. Certainly the interferon mechanism, having a wide spectrum of antiviral activity, offers some real hope for the control of viral infections.

Several factors determine the effective role of interferon in any particular infection: First, cells of the body must be available to respond by forming interferon; second, the capacity of the infecting virus to turn off the body cell which is vital to the production of interferon and its action; third, the degree of stimulation exerted by the virus in provoking the interferon response; and finally, the sensitivity of the cells to respond to interferon and the sensitivity of the virus to the action of interferon. The interferon mechanism appears to be very complicated; the end result depends not only on the production of interferon, but also on the virus, and the ability of the cells to produce interferon.

Interferon has been demonstrated in acute viral infections in the serum of the blood and in washings from the nose of patients with the common cold and in the saliva of patients with mumps. Interferon when injected into the veins lasts but a few minutes. In the research laboratory, mice previously infected with tuberculosis produced interferon after intravenous injection with tuberculin whereas the injection of tuberculin in noninfected mice failed to cause an interferon response. Immune systems of the body are interrelated and the substances that interfere with antibodies may also interfere with the production of interferon. X-ray radiation, steroids, and other toxic agents may also interfere with the production of interferon. A substance known as BCG has been found to promote the production of antibody and interferon. Certain drugs known to suppress the immune response may not affect interferon production.

Effective antiviral treatment is greatly needed by the medical profession to control such diseases as hepatitis, various forms of encephalitis and other crippling illnesses. A major problem at the present time is the production of sufficient quantities of effective interferon for the treat-

ment of patients. Intensive study is being carried out
to develop methods of producing sufficient quantities
of human interferon. The amounts of pure and potent human
interferon available have greatly limited studies on patients.
In conclusion, interferon is an intrinsic part of the host's
ability to resist injury from viruses and many other germs.
There is hope that resistance of host cells may be stimulated
by the interferon system and permit further study of interferon's therapeutic application to infectious and oncological
diseases such as cancer.

Chapter 10

EPILOGUE

IT APPEARS THAT *multiple sclerosis* is exactly what the name implies: a disease of many scars causally related to common virus infections occurring most often in childhood. MS is complex because the brain is very complex, made up of many essential and vital organs. The symptoms and signs of MS are variable with many "ups" and "downs." Common childhood diseases are caused by different viruses, many of which may cause inflammation of the brain and spinal cord as a complication or aftereffect. This complicating disease is called acute encephalomyelitis. The term might be applied to the acute form of MS. When remissions and exacerbations occur the disease is diagnosed as MS. Dr. Ludo Van Bogaert (1950) described four of nineteen cases of acute encephalomyeltiis which later developed the classical symptoms and signs of multiple sclerosis.

Viruses of common childhood diseases in particular are known to cause acute encephalomyelitis. The changes in the brain cells are similar to those found in the chronic form of scarred or demyelinated areas in the brain designated as *plaques*. A final definition of MS could be multiple scars from previous acute encephalomyelitis. The symptoms and signs often begin with inflammation of the optic nerve or portions of the body involving half of the limbs, one arm or leg or all four limbs. When the optic nerve is inflamed and the spinal cord also becomes inflamed the disease is designated neuromyelitis optica. This is a form of acute encephalomyelitis which is very acute and severe with a high mortality. It occurs in its most acute form in children and complete survival rarely occurs or the process leads to death within a few months or a year.

The diagnosis of acute encephalomyelitis is based on scattered signs of involvement of the nervous system very similar to those seen in the chronic form of MS. Encephalomyelitis rarely follows a vaccination with live virus such as the vaccinia virus; or it may folow infectious diseases such as chicken pox, rubella or the simple common Herpes virus infection often referred to as a cold sore or fever blister proved to be caused by the Herpes virus. Other common childhood diseases such as colds or mumps on occasion cause encephalitis but do not cause serious demyelination as is known to be associated with rubeola or measles virus. The latter cause inflammation of the brain years after childhood measles diagnosed subacute sclerosing panencephalitis (SSPE). The chronic form of measles encephalitis is occasionally referred to as disseminated or multiple sclerosis.

It was a hundred years ago that Jean Martin Charcot recorded the classical symptoms and signs of multiple sclerosis, which he stated were *tremor* and *nystagmus*. The third symptom which he elaborated was a hesitant or slow jerky-type of talking, which he called *scanning speech.* Charcot described concisely the injury to the brain considered classic pathologic changes seen by the microscope after the patient has passed away. He pointed out that the coverings of the nerves were destroyed, and he called this demyelination or lack of myelin.

While the symptoms of MS may develop in childhood it is relatively uncommon, and most often symptoms begin between the ages of twenty and forty years.

Measles is one of the oldest and most important diseases of mankind. In English it is known as *rubeola* and should not be confused with rubella as these virus diseases are entirely different and distinct. Measles was suspected of being a virus disease early in the twentieth century, but it was not until Enders and Peebles (1954) were successful in isolating the virus from throat washings of patients who were early in the eruptive phase of their disease that the virus cause of measles was proved. Measles virus is included among the myxoviruses along with Newcastle disease virus, influenza viruses and distemper virus in dogs and minks, and a disease in cattle called rinderpest.

The measles, distemper and rinderpest viruses are interrelated, and they all represent the same virus in their respective hosts, humans, dogs, and cattle. A very serious complication of measles is measles encephalitis. Viruses isolated from brain tissue studied by the light and electron microscope have shapes identical with those shown caused by proved measles virus infection in tissue cultured cells.

Before the measles vaccine became available in 1963 over 400 deaths a year occurred from measles in the United States. The death rate has been sharply reduced coincident with the use of the live measles vaccine which causes a mild case of measles, sometimes a low fever and occasionally a rash, but the patient develops protective antibodies which probably provide lifetime immunity. The long-range consequences or aftereffects of the live measles vaccine are still unknown. Although SSPE may occur five to twenty years after childhood measles, the most chronic aftereffects of the vaccine are as yet unknown.

MS on occasion is a mild or benign disease and may remain silent for years or forever. The degree of involvement varies widely and in a small proportion of patients doubt about the presence of MS exists because of the lack of any clear symptoms or signs. Changes in the eyes, such as pallor of the discs, may suggest possible MS. Patients in the doubtful or probable category have higher measles antibodies in their blood or spinal fluid. The term "Unrestricted" refers to patients who have no restriction of activity for normal employment or domestic purposes, but they are not necessarily symptom free. There is a group of patients with MS referred to as "Clinically silent" and only discovered to have MS at autopsy. In a few rare and exceptional cases the disease is permanently arrested. Some patients remain in perfect health for months or years.

Early symptoms are elicited after very careful inquiry dating back even into childhood. The early symptoms relate to visual difficulty or even double vision, weakness in an arm or leg with some difficulty in walking or numbness and tingling accompanied by double vision. Pain is rarely an early symptom, but it is often attributed to arthritis or rheumatism. Some blurring of vision occurs temporarily following physical exercise. A careful examination by an eye specialist will occasionally reveal optic neuritis. Symptoms and signs fluctuate and the majority of patients have definite periods when they are free or relieved of symptoms. These periods last for months or years. It is important to inform the patient about his illness and give reassurance regarding importance of remissions or periods of recovery many of which last a long time.

Patients with spinal cord disease are seriously ill and are in need of reassurance regarding emotional disturbances or family instability. When this has been accomplished the patient is prepared for reeducation in sexual as well as other areas. Interest in sex persists and should be discussed in a matter-of-fact way by the patient's own physician.

The distribution of MS in the world has led to an intensive search for clues to the possible cause of MS. The findings show there are regions in the world where the disease is more common than elsewhere with high and low frequency areas. In general they are the cold and hot regions of the world, being highest in the colder and the low in the warmest places such as the tropics. Measles is worldwide and like MS and poliomyelitis is recognized as involving the nervous system more commonly in the colder regions of the world. Measles encephalitis, the most serious form of the disease, is rare in Africa and tropical climates. The measles and polio viruses are grouped together by virologists. They are both found in the nose and throat and in the bowels of man. The changes caused by these viruses are distinct and different. Paralysis in poliomyelitis is mainly of the motor nerves to the legs and arms. Weakness and paralysis in measles encephalitis is manifest by involvement of the brain and spinal cord itself. Blindness or loss of vision in measles is due to injury to the optic tracts in the brain. Optic neuritis is common in association with measles encephalitis and many patients with optic neuritis eventually develop signs of MS. In the northern hemisphere high risk regions are found in Europe or in places colonized by the Europeans. Epidemiologists recognize that we are dealing with a rare disease and the diagnosis is based on clinical signs. So, meaningful prevalence rates are certainly subject to error. At this time there is no perfect study on the frequency of multiple sclerosis.

Recent research in multiple sclerosis has been concerned with genetic factors, and certain HL-A antigens are found increased in patients with MS. Patients with high measles antibodies carry HLA-3, 7 and/or 18, suggesting that genetic factors contribute to the control of antibody production. Geneticists find that LD7a is a genetic determinant which occurs in 60 to 70 percent of patients with multiple sclerosis. It is known that measles antibodies tend to be higher in MS patients than in controls, but persons who bear HLA-3 have higher measles antibody titers than those who do not, whether they have MS or not. It has been suggested by some investigators that the occurrence of measles late in childhood might increase the likelihood of acquiring MS. The investigators emphasize the difficulties of evaluating any form of treatment.

Immunologists have been studying the results of transfer factor in patients with MS. A selective suppression of measles virus was present in some patients with MS, and it was this selective depression which prompted the investigation of transfer factor and the ability of cells in the body to react to measles virus. Fifteen patients were studied and eleven developed significantly higher values of measles virus following the use of transfer factor. Sixteen patients inoculated with transfer factor at weekly intervals exhibited an increase in their response to measles virus.

A virus disease called *Visna* is a chronic inflammatory demyelinating disease of the central nervous system of sheep. Although visna has no counterpart in human beings, sheep may provide an animal model to study persistence of virus having potential application in the study of multiple sclerosis.

The pathologic findings in mature dogs with ODE strongly support a relationship to MS, SSPE and Neuromyelitis Optica in human beings. ODE is a valuable animal model for further study of severe demyelinating diseases in dogs and man.

The relationship between measles antibodies and oligoclonal immune globulin in spinal fluid of patients with MS recorded that measles virus antibodies occurred in the serum and spinal fluid of more than 80 percent of patients with MS. Patients with MS were compared with patients with SSPE proved due to measles virus. In patients with SSPE the immune globulin represents an oligoclonal response to a high level of antibody against the measles virus.

Brain material from patients with multiple sclerosis has been studied with the electron microscope and pictures are similar to those occurring in association with cells proved to be infected by measles virus.

In considering prevention and treatment of disease it is important to recognize how we defend ourselves against invaders such as viruses. Viruses persist in the body of infected persons in spite of the fact that we have antibodies against the particular virus concerned. There are several well-known examples of persistent viral infections in man. One is the virus of the common cold sore, Herpes virus, and the closely related cytomegalovirus. The immune systems of the body are responsible for checking the destructive ability of viruses and on occasion are responsible for manifestations of an infection. A virus spreads from one cell to another when cells are multiplying or dividing. A mechanism of immunity called "cellular-immunity" consists of cells such as lymphocytes and plasma cells which produce a lymphotoxin or interferon, a protein substance which inhibits or prevents a virus from multiplying and thus could prevent other cells from becoming infected. Certain cells in the body make interferon much better than other cells. Viruses infect cells of the immune system such as in leukemia and thus depress the immune response. One approach to treating chronically infected individuals is to induce the production of interferon. The basic cell of the immune system works through the thymus gland to produce certain types of lymphocytes known to the immunologist as "T" cells. Some work through the bone marrow to produce another type of immune cell known as "B" lymphocytes. Antibodies formed in the body do not cause recovery from infection but they help to prevent getting disease a second or third time. The principal role of the immune system is prevention. Treatment must be considered in terms of prevention. Smallpox, poliomyelitis and measles are prevented by inoculating individuals with a safe and modified form of virus. Although the primary approach to treatment is prevention, the possibility of stimulating the immune mechanisms is under intensive study. A remission or relief from the symptoms in patients with multiple sclerosis may last for months and even years. This certainly lends hope to the fact that the immune systems can be encouraged and induced either to produce a period of recovery or a remission.

Interferon discovered in 1957 has proved to be a defense mechanism of importance in recovery from acute and sometimes chronic infections. Interferon may be the major determinant in recovery from illness because it interferes with the multiplication of viruses. It not only arrests the multiplication and spread of viruses, but is active in the actual destruction of viruses in the prevention of reinfection. The name implies interference with the processes of development such as cancer, where the effects of interferon are also under intensive investigation. Interferon is not in itself directly antiviral but produces an effect against viruses and cells by inducing the formation of a new substance which activates the antiviral mechanism. Interferon is thought to act by two mechanisms. First, to stimulate the production of another substance which is directly antiviral, and second, to work in combination with cell components to produce an antiviral state. The important role of antibody is prevention, and it is questionable whether antibody is effective after the viral infection has become established. Most experimental evidence supports a direct relationship between the interferon system and recovery from infections. The control of virus disease may be approached first by prevention through the development of vaccines, and second, control by chemical means employing certain substances which have antiviral activity, such as idoxuridine which has been shown to have an antiviral effect against Herpes viruses. The interferon mechanism having a wide range of antiviral activity offers some real hope for the control of viral infections. A major problem at present exists in the production of sufficient quantities of effective interferon for treatment of patients. Amounts of pure and potent interferon available have greatly limited experimental studies on patients. Interferon is an intrinsic part of the host's ability to resist injury from viruses and many other germs.

Finally, what are some of the answers on the horizon for MS? Prospectives for earlier diagnostic procedures are bright, making possible earlier treatment and stabilization of the scarring process in MS. The value of such diagnostic tests are under intensive study.* Animal models such as mice, sheep and dogs are in the experimental laboratory. The antibiotic era is making way for the antiviral era. New antiviral agents offer hopeful prospects for better control and prevention of the basic causes of MS.

---

* Editorial: Virus Markers in Multiple Sclerosis, *New England Journal of Medicine,* June 24, 1976.

SELECTED READING

Millar, J.H.D., M.D., F.R.C.P. *Multiple Sclerosis, A Disease Acquired in Childhood,* 1971 Charles C Thomas, Springfield, Illinois, U.S.A.

Davis, M.Z., R.N., D.N.S. *Living with Multiple Sclerosis,* 1973 Charles C Thomas, Springfield, Illinois, U.S.A.

McAlpine, Douglas, Lumsden, C.E., Acheson, E.D., *Multiple Sclerosis, A Reappraisal,* 1972 Churchill Livingstone, London, England.

Leibowitz, U. and associates. Epidemiological study of multiple sclerosis in Israel. *J. Neurol. Neurosurg. Psychiat. 29*:60-68, 1966.

Baron, S. and Isaacs, A. Mechanism of recovery from viral infections in the chick embryo. *Nature, 191*:97-98, 1961.

Kurtzke, J. F. A Reassessment of the distribution of multiple sclerosis. Parts I and II. *Acta Neurol. Scandinav. 51*:110-157, 1975.

Greenblatt, M.H. *Multiple Sclerosis and Me,* 1972 Charles C Thomas, Springfield, Illinois, U.S.A.

Stanley, W.M. and Valens, E.G. *Viruses and the Nature of Life,* 1961 E.P. Dutton & Co. Inc., New York, U.S.A.

Alter, M., and Kurtzke, J. F. (Eds.): *The Epidemiology of Multiple Sclerosis.* 1968, Charles C Thomas, Springfield, Illinois, U.S.A.

Rose, A. S. and associates: Co-operative study in evaluation of therapy in multiple sclerosis: ACTH vs placebo, *Neurology,* 20:2, 1, 1970.

GLOSSARY, DEFINITIONS

Explanation of Terms

ACTH: Abbreviation for adrenocorticotrophic hormone; no basis for use of ACTH as a long-term treatment for MS patients.

ANTIBODIES: Substances produced by cells in response to stimulating agents such as viruses or bacteria. They are quite *specific* in their ability to protect against infection—that is, polio antibodies will protect against poliomyelitis only.

ANTIGEN: A molecular protein substance such as a virus; antigens stimulate an "immune response."

ASTROCYTE: A type of brain cell.

ATAXIA: Failure of muscular coordination.

AUTOPSY: Examination of a body after death.

BENIGN: Not malignant, favorable for recovery.

B-CELLS: Make proteins known as "immunoglobulins."

BCG: Stands for Bacillus Calmette-Guerin, a strain of tuberculosis bacterium.

CELL: The body is made up almost entirely of many different kinds of cells. Each cell has a discrete inner core called the nucleus, surrounded by cytoplasm, and is encased in a membrane separating it from other cells.

CELLULAR IMMUNOLOGY: One of the body's immune systems.

CEREBROSPINAL FLUID (CSF): Fluid surrounding the brain and spinal cord.

CLINICAL: Pertaining to the actual observation and treatment of *patients,* as distinguished from theoretical or experimental observations.

67

COMPLEMENT: A substance in serum that combines with antigen-antibody complex. Symbol C'.

DEMYELINATION: Destruction or removal of the myelin covering nerve tissue.

DEVIC'S DISEASE: See Neuromyelitis optica.

DIAGNOSIS: The art of distinguishing one disease from another.

DISC: Disk, a thin circular object in the back of the eyeball.

DISSEMINATED: Scattered or distributed (multiple).

DISTEMPER: An infectious disease of animals related to rubeola in man.

EAE: Experimental allergic encephalomyelitis, induced in animals by *basic protein* of myelin.

ELECTRON MICROSCOPE: Powered by a unit of negative electricity, capable of magnifying several 100,000 times.

ENCEPHALITIS: Inflammation of the brain, sometimes called "sleeping sickness" caused by viruses and other microscopic organisms.

EPIDEMIOLOGY: The science concerned with the cause, frequency, and distribution of an infectious process or a physiological state in a human community.

ETIOLOGY: The study of the *causes* of diseases.

EXACERBATION: Increase in severity of any symptom or disease.

EXOGENOUS: Originating outside the organism.

GAMMA GLOBULIN: A protein fraction of the blood serum which is known to contain many different kinds of antibodies.

GENETIC DETERMINANT: Pertaining to heredity, i.e. HL-A antigen.

IODODEOXYURIDINE: A drug useful in the treatment of Herpes virus infections. Abr. I.D.U.

IMMUNITY: Security against any particular disease or poison, i.e. gamma globulin.

IMMUNE RESPONSES: Concern ridding the body of foreign substances.

INCLUSION BODY: Included within a cell, such as viral particles.

INTERFERON: An interfering substance that neutralizes viruses. It is produced by the body's cells in response to foreign nucleic acid, such as viruses. It protects un-infected cells.

LATENT: Concealed, or late appearing.

LESION: A loss of function of a part.

LEVAMISOLE: An immunopotentiating drug which re-stores the function of lymphocytes to normal.

LYMPHOCYTE: A variety of white blood cell related to the immune systems of the body. (See B and T cells.)

MICRON: A unit of measure in the metric system.

MYELIN: A substance which forms a covering or sheath around nerve fibers.

MYXOVIRUS: A virus which causes disease in mucous tissue, such as the throat, mouth or lung. (Influenza.)

NEURASTHENIA: Nervous exhaustion, characterized by abnormal fatigability.

NEURITIS: Inflammation of a nerve.

NEUROMYELITIS OPTICA: Acute transverse myelitis with optic neuritis.

NEURON: A nerve cell with its processes.

NYSTAGMUS: A rapid movement of the eyeball.

OLIGOCLONAL IMMUNE GLOBULIN: Protein anti-body from many immune forming cells.

ONCOLOGICAL: Related to cancer.

PARALYSIS AGITANS: A characteristic tremor of resting muscles.

PATHOLOGY: Deals with the essential nature of disease.

PLACEBO: An inactive substance used to determine the efficacy of medicinal substances, such as, ACTH.

PLAQUE: A patch or flat area, such as a scar.

PLASMA CELL: A blood cell related to immunity.

PREVALENCE RATE: The number of cases present in a given community at one time divided by the population of the community at the same time. Example: 7 cases/ 350 people in the town.

REMISSION: diminution or abatement of symptoms.

RINDERPEST: A distemper-like disease of cattle, related to distemper in dogs.

RUBELLA: A disease with a measly-like rash, often called "three-day measles" or German measles, due to rubella virus. It is not measles.

RUBEOLA: Regular or common measles with blotchy rash, cough, running nose, and inflamed eyes, due to rubeola virus.

SCANNING SPEECH: Recurrent pauses, jerky speech.

SCAR: Sclerotic or demyelinated area in brain.

SEQUELA: A condition following or caused by a previous disease; an aftereffect of illness.

SLOW VIRUS: A term used to indicate persistence or latency causing disease months or years after the initial illness.

SSPE: Subacute sclerosing panencephalitis, a severe demyelinating disease of the brain caused by the measles virus.

TISSUE CLUTURE: Living tissue cells growing in special solutions conducive to their growth, usually in glass tubes or bottles.

SCLEROSIS: Hard, such as a scar or plaque.

T-CELLS: Constitute a "cell-mediated" immune response.

TITER: A level, or strength of a substance such as antibodies in serum.

TRANSFER FACTOR: A substance which stimulates the immune system to increase its activity.

TRANSVERSE MYELITIS: Inflammation of the spinal cord.

VACCINIA: A virus disease of cattle. A virus used to vaccinate against smallpox.

VIRUS: A living agent, the smallest and simplest form of life, which depends on other living cells in order to replicate or reproduce itself. From the *Oxford English Dictionary*, 1778: "Venice is a stink-pot, charged with the very virus of hell!" Prior to the ending of the nineteenth century, *virus* was known as a foul, offensive, poisonous fluid. In 1892, Iwanowski, a Russian first reported the results of filtration experiments (keeping out bacteria) with tobacco-mosaic disease. Independently, a Dutchman, Beijerinck, in 1898 repeated the same experiment. He realized that a new type of infectious agent, which he called *contagium vivum fluidum,* had been discovered.

INDEX

73